THIS NOTEBOOK BELONGS TO:

Made in the USA
Coppell, TX
18 December 2022

90098311R00069